# TAKE CONTROL
# OF YOUR
# BACK PAIN

# TAKE CONTROL
# OF YOUR
# BACK PAIN

## Learn How To STOP Hurting Yourself, AND Take CONTROL of Your Pain

## Matthew Michaels MD

**Limit of Liability Disclaimer:** The information contained in this book is for information purposes only, and may not apply to your situation. The author, publisher, distributor, and provider provide no warranty about the content or accuracy of content enclosed. Information provided is subjective. Keep this in mind when reviewing this guide.

Although the author and publisher have made every effort to ensure that the information in this book was correct at press time, the author and publisher do not assume and hereby disclaim any liability to any party for any loss, damage, or disruption caused by errors or omissions, whether such errors or omissions result from negligence, accident, or any other cause.

This book is not intended as a substitute for the medical advice. The reader should regularly consult a physician in matters relating to his/her health and particularly with respect to any symptoms that may require diagnosis or medical attention.

It's important to understand that catastrophic things do occur. Although the odds are low, it's possible that your musculoskeletal pain is a result of infection, tumor, or other unusual pathology that requires medical attention. It's also possible that your back pain issue might fall into the small percentage of cases with unusual characteristics that won't respond to this paradigm. The only way to be sure you're not experiencing one of the above is to see a physician for diagnosis. If your pain doesn't promptly respond to the advice given here within 2 weeks, I strongly advise you to see an interventional physical medicine and rehabilitation specialist as soon as possible.

This book is not intended to be a didactic review of the science of low back pain. It's meant to be used by you, the reader, as a tool to help you understand your pain, to treat it independently as much as possible, and to gain insights into the working of the medical system as it relates to back pain.

**Website:** www.whydoIhavebackpain.com
**Email:** tri3md@gmail.com
**Phone:** 503 535 8302

Ordering Information: Quantity sales. Special discounts are available on multiple purchases by corporations, associations, and others.

For details, contact the "Special Sales Department" at the address above.

Matthew Michaels MD —1st edition, 2017

Book Layout: © 2016 EvolveGlobalPublishing.com

ISBN: (Paperback) 978-1-945604-17-1
ISBN: (Hardcover) 978-1-945604-27-0
ISBN-13: (Createspace) 978-1974374144
ISBN-10: (Createspace) 19743/4149
ISBN: (Smashwords) 9781370214235
ASIN: (Amazon Kindle) B071GQ4FB4

This book is available on Barnes & Noble, Kobo, Apple iBooks (digital)

# Table of Contents

# About The Author

Matthew Michaels is a #1 internationally best-selling American author, he's a successful Medical Doctor, board certified in Physical Medicine and Rehabilitation.

As a clinician, Dr. Michaels' main work is at RestorePDX in Beaverton, Oregon. Dr. Michaels' focus is on painful conditions of the Musculoskeletal and Neurologic systems. He has developed a specific system of integration of treatment with specially qualified and like-minded physical therapists, and chiropractors. These professionals understand that therapy should involve an intensive process of evaluation for musculoskeletal imbalance and motion dysfunction and that the primary long term treatment of these conditions should focus on education for modification of posture and behavior.

Dr. Michaels has a passion for helping his patients, and the medical community as a whole, come to understand that the real solution for these painful conditions comes from giving you, the patient, an intimate knowledge of exactly why you are having pain. That the ultimate cure comes from insight and knowledge giving you the power to help yourself, rather than from someone else doing something to you.

Dr. Michaels spends a great deal of time and effort developing professional networks that work in an interdisciplinary fashion. These networks involve therapists who understand how best to use the skills of their Allopathic and Osteopathic colleagues, and Physicians who know how best to integrate their skills into a comprehensive rehabilitation program.

Dr. Michaels earned his MD at The Medical College of Virginia at Virginia Commonwealth University from 1988-1992, and graduated AOA and Phi Kappa Phi in 1992.

Dr. Michaels completed a transitional residency program at Roanoke Memorial Hospital in 1993.

Dr. Michaels trained for his specialty in Physical Medicine and Rehabilitation from 1993-1996 at The University of Colorado Health Sciences Center in Denver, Colorado.

Dr. Michaels became a Diplomate of the American Board of Physical Medicine and Rehabilitation, and a Fellow of the American Academy of Physical Medicine and Rehabilitation in 1997.

Dr. Michaels became a Diplomate of the American Board of Electrodiagnostic Medicine in 1997.

Dr. Michaels has been practicing Interventional Physiatry since 1996. He is currently practicing at RestorePDX in Beaverton, Oregon

One of the main reasons Matthew chose Interventional Physiatry is due to a lengthy history of Chronic Low back pain and sciatica. Dr. Michaels found all current systems of back pain treatment to be inadequate as they could only really help modestly with current flare ups while doing nothing about the frequent re-occurences that tend to lead to progressive disability. This frustration led Dr. Michaels to his current system of treatment focusing on the prevention of disabling flare-ups of pain.

Dr. Michaels' practice has evolved into treatment of the most chronic and complex of musculoskeletal and neurologic problems. This focus allows him to see through the diagnostic haze to better identify the underlying biomechanical cause of pain so he can treat the actual problem rather than just the symptom.

Dr. Michaels lives in NW Portland. He is a competitive triathlete having completed numerous Sprint and Olympic distance races as well multiple IM 70.3 events, and Ironman Arizona in 2012. You will find him running the Portland trails with his two German Shepherd dogs in summer and skiing the glades in winter.

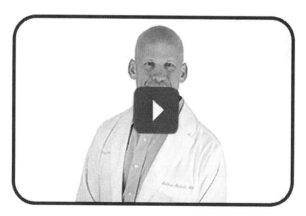

For **Free Video Information**
On This Subject Go To
***whydoihavebackpain.com***

# Introduction

I finished my training in physical medicine and rehabilitation in 1996. I was 31 years old at my graduation, and I'd been experiencing back and sciatic nerve pain for 19 years.

I saw an orthopedic surgeon for my first episode of back pain when I was 12 — a visit which led to a diagnosis of sciatica and nothing else. He had no advice and nothing to offer. For most of the following years, I experienced frequent and at times disabling flare-ups.

When I was 20, I went on a two-week vacation to the Caribbean and had such intense back pain that I spent 10 days nearly immobile in the hotel room. I went to see a physical therapist on the island, who gave me some ideas regarding how to resolve my pain. These ideas involved primarily McKenzie-type extension exercises, which did in fact help but didn't solve the problem.

At times, the pain was so intense I thought I might never again live a normal life. Despite that, I enjoyed periods of relative ease during which I exercised consistently.

Since 1996, I've been practicing in the field of interventional physical medicine and rehabilitation. During residency and for years thereafter, I trained extensively to become an interventional pain management doctor, focusing primarily on interventional procedures.

As I dealt with my own pain and that of my patients, I began to develop a better understanding of the role of physical therapy and behavior modification, which enabled me to see more success over time in the treatment of both my patients and myself. At first, I became enamored with the special skills of manual physiotherapists — but I later came to view those manual skills as no more valuable than injection techniques, as they're passive tools that can't really change the underlying issues.

As time went by, I started to notice patterns in my own pain flare-ups. That, combined with my understanding of the underlying anatomy and injuries involved, helped me develop the process presented in this book.

The early versions of the process started with sending patients to McKenzie therapy, where I saw mixed success that nonetheless was better than any other kind of physical therapy. I then began to notice that my posture had a major impact on my pain reproduction and that simple things, like the way I brushed my teeth or washed the dishes, could also cause or reduce the flare-ups.

I also began to notice that when I told people to avoid the behavioral issues that always led to my own flare-ups, they'd often return to my office for a follow-up and tell me they felt much better. I'd naturally assume their improvements were a result of following my orders and seeking physical therapy intervention, but they'd frequently say things like, "I never went to therapy! I simply did what you told me to do, and the pain went away."

This began a transition in my practice. During the first visit, I began to carefully review the patient's posture and behaviors and to give advice regarding how to change these elements. I then selected local physical therapists who would follow my orders: to focus more on instructing the patient regarding behavior and posture than on exercise or on manipulating or adjusting the spine.

This led to much greater success for my patients with back and other types of pain. I found my patients required less intervention, less medication, and fewer injections — and that they in fact fared much better over time.

In this book, I present the theory of movement and behavior that I've just described. The following chapters will discuss the nature of low back pain and how it should best be treated — not with pills, injections, or surgery, but with behavior modification guided by a better understanding of what's actually going on in the spine.

This work represents a distillation of 21 years of medical practice in the field of interventional pain management in chronic musculoskeletal pain, as well as 40 years of personal experience with chronic low back pain. It's dedicated to my patients and to anyone else who needs a little extra help to control similar pain and to get back on track. I hope you find it useful.

DISCLAIMER: It's important to understand that catastrophic things do occur. Although the odds are low, it's possible that your musculoskeletal pain is a result of infection, tumor, or other unusual pathology that requires medical attention. It's also possible that your back pain issue might fall into the small percentage of cases with unusual characteristics that won't respond to this paradigm or that could cause a disabling loss of neurologic function. The only way to be sure you're not experiencing one of the above is to see a physician for diagnosis. If you are experiencing loss of or decrease in bowel or bladder control, if you are experiencing loss of strength in your legs, or loss of balance or if your pain doesn't promptly respond to the advice given here within 2 weeks, I strongly advise you to see an interventional physical medicine and rehabilitation specialist as soon as possible.

This book is not intended to be a didactic review of the science of low back pain. It's meant to be used by you, the reader, as a tool to help you understand your pain, to treat it independently as much as possible, and to gain insights into the working of the medical system as it relates to back pain.

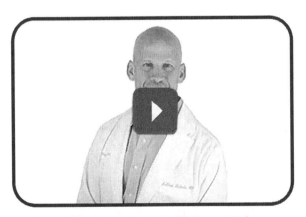

For **Free Video Information**
On This Subject Go To
*whydoihavebackpain.com*

# Why do I have back pain?

The following factors are critical to helping you through chronic back pain. They apply not only to this current episode of pain but also to future episodes, and will help you to understand how to deal with and minimize them. In these chapters, you'll learn:

- The real problem causing your pain. How your lifestyle, posture, and behavior will collectively impact your future with this pain. What you should avoid doing each day. What you should start doing each day to protect your spine.
- The role of range of motion, strength, and flexibility exercises. The role of aerobic exercise. The roles that physical therapy and/or chiropractic treatment can and should play.
- The role that injection techniques can and should play. The role that surgical intervention can and should play. The emerging role of regenerative interventions (potential game-changer).

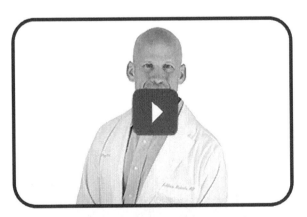

For **Free Video Information**
On This Subject Go To
***whydoihavebackpain.com***

# CHAPTER 1

# Understand the real problem causing your pain

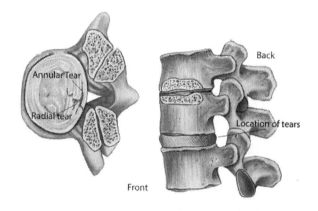

*Figure 1: The primary source of all back pain: tears in the posterior annulus fibrosis*

## CASE STUDY #1: Discogenic pain in a patient who's been to physical therapy and thinks more therapy won't help him

BP is a 50-year-old man who came to my office with chronic low back pain. He was in the midst of an intense flare-up and requesting urgent help.

He'd been to physical therapy many times in the past and felt he had nothing new to learn, so he wasn't interested in my sending him for the specialized physical therapy that I knew would help him. He specifically requested that I perform an injection to settle his pain — and given that he refused to go to therapy and that the circumstances indicated he'd likely respond to injection, I agreed.

He underwent a right-sided L5 and S1 transforaminal epidural steroid injection (an injection of local anesthetic and a small amount of cortisone through the spinal nerve opening at the level that hurt), and he had a dramatic response. His pain resolved virtually completely within a day or two. Upon follow-up, he was thrilled with his outcome. But once again, he refused to go to physical therapy as he felt he'd already done it and wouldn't benefit from more.

Two months later, I got a call from him at 2:00am on a Sunday. He'd been out picnicking that day and somehow hurt his back again. He was miserable. He couldn't sleep and could barely move. I advised him to lie on the floor on his belly (either flat or propped up on his elbows) for the next half-hour, trying to gently arch his back into the pain. I also advised him to come into my office first thing in the morning.

When I saw him, he was doing significantly better. He could move properly, but his spine was still forward-flexed and shifted to the side. It seemed he'd finally seen the light, as he was responsive to my suggestion to undergo physical therapy. Over the course of the next two months, he learned the behavior-modification program that I've outlined in this book. His back pain has been significantly better ever since.

## Case study #2: Chronic recurrent discogenic low back pain that only resolved with advice

JL is a 40-year-old male who came to my office with his third episode of low back pain.

He described his pain as a 7/10 and stated that it prevented him from doing anything fun after work. His previous episodes of pain had all lasted roughly two to three weeks, and this current episode was into its sixth week. He told me he was interested in doing whatever he possibly could to get rid of this current pain and to prevent future episodes.

During the evaluation, he had all the classic signs of a lumbar disc injury. I gave him advice regarding his posture and suggested he should change his approach to everyday activities such as washing the dishes, cooking dinner, running the vacuum cleaner, making the bed, brushing his teeth, etc. I referred him for appropriate physical therapy and suggested he should follow up with me in four weeks. He was also advised that if physical therapy was overly painful, he should follow up more rapidly so we could take action to settle the pain — preventing him from wasting his time in physical therapy.

Four weeks later, he presented to my office telling my medical assistant that his pain was completely resolved. I assumed that physical therapy had done the trick for him and asked him how he liked the physical therapist. He laughed a little and said, "Doc, I never met the therapist! I just changed the way I did everyday things, and the pain went away."

For the most part, lower back pain is very simple to understand if you start by accepting that the lumbar disc is at the heart of virtually all of it. (For now, we'll ignore the possibility of more severe and complex types of pathology and focus on more common types of back pain, which aren't life-threatening or potentially permanently disabling.)

Some of us may be unlucky enough to be born with fragile discs or sub-optimal spinal curvature (like me), so that even at a very young age, the lumbar disc may show a greater propensity for injury. But even for the average person, back pain is among the most common musculoskeletal pain complaints — and since the vast majority of low back pain is related to a disc injury, we know that even normal discs are prone to a particular type of injury.

The anatomy of the disc, which allows it to perform its biomechanical function, also makes it susceptible to injury.

The disc is made up of concentric rings of cartilage called the annulus fibrosis (AF) and a soft cushioning center called the nucleus pulposus (NP).

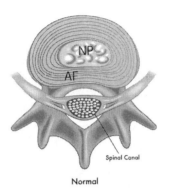

Normal

*Figure 2: The AF forms the semi-flexible union between vertebral bodies and is filled in the center by a contained gelatinous cushion (the NP).*

As a result of our anatomy and our behavior, the back of the AF is very prone to injury.

Here's what happens: as we bend forward, the back-third to back-half of the AF stretches while the front compresses. This creates a major pressure gradient, squeezing the NP towards the stretched and weakened backside of the disc, where it can eventually tear through the AF. These tears (even small ones) are exquisitely painful — and as the tears extend further backward, they cause pain that radiates from the center of the spine toward the buttock and eventually all the way down the leg.

Beyond the mechanical effects of tears of the AF, the chemical nature of the NP causes inflammation when it touches anything other than the pocket of the AF in which it's supposed to stay. So as soon as the NP moves outside that home base, it causes intense swelling and irritation. This tearing and subsequent inflammatory reaction then leads to muscle spasms, which can be excruciatingly painful.

The tears in the AF are referred to as radial (through the layers of annulus) and annular (between the layers of annulus). In addition to being the primary cause of disc degeneration, they're at the heart of all low back pain. The problem is made significantly worse by the fact that essentially all modern life places the lumbar spine in a flexed position, putting us at risk for acute tears or extension and worsening of chronic tears.

The intervertebral disc is, for most people, fragile and prone to injury. The biomechanics of modern life make the problem worse, but **it's actually our reaction to these injuries that leads to the chronic pain that so many people experience.**

As a rule, all people react to disc injury by leaning away from the pain. This is an automatic, instinctive reaction to the intense pain caused by the tear and by any pressure placed on the tear by allowing the vertebral end-plates to compress it. This automatic impulse to lean away almost always makes the pain better temporarily — but it also always makes the underlying problem worse.

The fluidity and flexibility of the disc, which allows our spines to bend and twist, also causes further injury. As we lean away from the pain, we put pressure on the part of the disc directly opposite the location of the tear. This creates high pressure opposite the tear and low pressure at the tear, driving yet more NP into the tear.

**It's critical to remember that as you seek comfort by leaning away from the pain, you'll feel better temporarily while actually making the problem worse.** This is why so many people with low back pain complain that they can find a comfortable position while sitting to watch a movie or to eat a meal but that standing straight is even more painful afterwards.

In this way lower back pain feeds on itself, is exacerbated and becomes chronic. Keep in mind that **your body's reflexive response to low back pain is always the wrong thing to do.**

After reading this book, you'll notice people who are clearly kinked or leaning to one side. These people look for all the world as though one leg is shorter than the other — but leg-length discrepancies are very unusual without some prior trauma to one leg. Just imagine the impact that chronically leaning to one side (because of an old back injury) will have on your future with back pain.

The solution is to understand that one should never let low back pain force you to lean away from the pain. Although it's counter-intuitive, you must in fact make the pain temporarily worse in order to get better faster or to get better at all.

In your mind, you should visualize your back pain as a tear in your back where you hurt the most. It doesn't matter if that's central or on the right or left side. As you sit, stand, and move, do your best to put pressure on the tear by standing up straight and pushing your body into the pain — into the straightest alignment you can achieve. This will close the open mouth of the tear, creating high pressure at the tear and low pressure opposite the tear. By intentionally creating this pressure gradient you'll allow the nucleus material to retreat back inside the pocket of the disc, where it should be.

Everything will change regarding your present and future back pain once you understand these very basic facts — that the lumbar disc is at the heart of all back pain and that leaning away from your pain will feel better at first, but will always make things worse in the long run — and once you act on this knowledge.

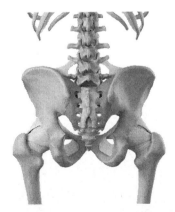

*Figure 3: Sacroiliac joint (in red)*

Other factors can play a role in back pain, but they're secondary. The facet joints and the sacroiliac joints can certainly play a role, but it's uncommon for them to become painful without an underlying disc problem. The sacroiliac joints and facet joints generally factor into back pain because of disc degeneration or the reflexive tendency to lean away from the pain (antalgic shift), creating asymmetry and asymmetrical degeneration of these joints. It's also important to know that the muscular pain associated with most back pain is usually spasm due to disc injury. It's rarely primary muscular pain.

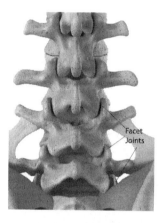

*Figure 4: Lumbar facet joints*

(A peculiar location of a disc tear within the nerve root opening or foramen can make the problem respond abnormally, where leaning into the pain reduces back pain but increases leg pain. This is difficult to resolve on your own, so you should seek medical attention in this circumstance.)

Unfortunately, the problem can get more insidious. Every tear leads to progressive loss of disc hydration and, eventually, to loss of disc height. Even worse, the tears tend to be asymmetrical or off-center. This means that the eventual collapse of the disc is also asymmetrical or off-center, leading to progressive curvature of the spine that doctors refer to as degenerative scoliosis.

Still worse: since we all reflexively lean away from the pain to reduce the discomfort caused by standing straight, our behavior feeds into the problem. Again, while leaning away from the tear modestly and temporarily reduces pain, it actually makes the situation worse in a variety of ways. Let's summarize:

- Leaning away from the pain extends the tear by depressurizing the tear itself and over-pressurizing the opposite side. This pushes more NP into the tear, but you won't know it's happening until you try to stand up straight.
- Shifting away from the pain feeds into the asymmetry that leads to additional problems down the road.
- The pain from a disc can be so intense that the body eventually shuts down the area and stops moving through the disc completely.
- The disc cartilage receives no blood supply and therefore relies on movement for nutrition. As we stop moving through the injured area, the degeneration of the disc only accelerates.

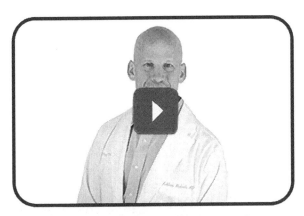

For **Free Video Information**
On This Subject Go To
***whydoihavebackpain.com***

# CHAPTER 2

# Gain an understanding of how your lifestyle, posture, and behavior will collectively impact your future with this pain

As we discussed, injuries to the backside of the lumbar disc are responsible for the majority of all low back pain. It's also important to understand that usually these injuries aren't sudden and acute; rather, they are the accumulation of minor injuries over the years that lead to progressively worsening disc tearing and pain.

Because modern life leads us to sit most of the time and to lean forward for almost all activities, we're nearly constantly placing stresses on the lumbar disc that promote injury. These stresses include everyday activities such as:

1. Sitting to relax.
2. Sitting to drive.
3. Leaning forward at the sink to do the dishes.
4. Prepping dinner ingredients at the counter.
5. Standing at the bathroom sink to brush your teeth.
6. Leaning into the mirror to better see yourself.
7. Loading the dishwasher.
8. Running the vacuum cleaner.
9. Making the bed.
10. Doing the laundry.

Any one of the above activities can cause a new episode of low back pain or a major flare-up for a chronic back pain sufferer.

The good news is that you can learn strategies to perform all these activities with better spinal alignment, in order to decrease harmful pressures within the lumbar disc. An understanding of the basic nature of lower back pain, and of how your posture, previous injuries, and behavior contribute to it, will make a major difference as the years go by.

Beyond modifying your everyday posture and behavior, among the most critical factors in maintaining your musculoskeletal health are movement and exercise. It's essential that you understand that all the connective tissues and cartilage have very poor blood flow. Yet strong, richly oxygenated blood flow is critical for maintaining tissue health and for repairing injury, so anything we can do to promote better flow will help prevent chronic injuries in the future.

Aerobic and graded resistance exercises are the best ways to promote better oxygenated blood flow and are critically important to maintaining musculoskeletal health. Virtually any form of exercise can induce abundant blood flow to most parts of the body and can promote better flow to those that are poorly supplied.

Joint lining (articular hyaline cartilage) and spinal discs (fibrocartilage) have essentially no blood supply and are nourished through movement. When these structures are compressed, fluid that's old, acidified, nutritionally depleted, and loaded with metabolic wastes is squeezed out. When the pressure is released, fluid is drawn back into the structures. In this way, hyaline and fibrocartilage essentially breathe. This breathing can only be induced by movement.

Furthermore, only those parts of any joint or structure that that are still moving properly are nourished. So when you sit or stand still, your cartilage is essentially starving and suffocating. And every day that goes by without you performing full range of motion causes your joints to lose further motion.

This process feeds on itself. The longer these structures go without moving, the more metabolic wastes accumulate, the longer this fluid sits still within the structures — the more it tends to drop in pH or become acidic. Acidic joint fluids are toxic to the cells that rebuild cartilage (chondroblasts). This means that **by sitting still, you're quite literally producing the conditions that will kill your cartilage and result in worsening arthritis.**

This process becomes a vicious cycle: sedentary behavior causes joint fluid to acidify, which leads to cartilage cell death, which leads to increasing pain, which leads to decreased movement, which leads to still more pain, and on and on. This applies to all your joints (hyaline or smooth cartilage) and the intervertebral discs (fibrocartilage).

I hope it's become abundantly clear that sedentary behavior is your enemy. Aerobic and range of motion exercises are your friends.

Put simply: you must keep moving. Loss of motion is generally both a major cause and a major consequence of most of the conditions we're discussing. It's for this reason that restoration of normal motion is the goal of our treatment.

Occasionally, we find structures that are painful due to too much motion (hypermobility). These conditions fall under special circumstances and will likely not respond well to the treatment plan presented here — yet another reason why you shouldn't follow these guidelines for more than two weeks if you're not seeing clear improvement. If this is the case, visit your local interventional physiatrist!

There is a misconception in modern society that exercise wears the body down and/or causes accelerated degeneration of the body. The opposite is true.

Perhaps one of the sources of this misconception is the notion that all exercise should subscribe to the "no pain, no gain" paradigm. Recent research confirms that exercise should be at least uncomfortable to be most effective, but it's most important to just get started with something fun and pleasant and to only push yourself harder when you've already developed the habit of exercise. Understanding this is important both for preventing injury and for helping the average person maintain an exercise habit.

It's true that exercise should be challenging and that your best gains will be made when it's at least somewhat unpleasant. But we have to recognize that the vast majority of people will tolerate very little in the way of discomfort, even when they know it's good for them. As such, it's important to recognize that any form of exercise is dramatically better than sedentary behavior.

I tell my patients that they must find some kind of exercise, activity, or effort they enjoy. Once they've developed a habit of exercise, and once exercise has become a part of their lives, only then do I recommend that they begin to accept the challenge of pushing themselves a little harder.

But for the chronic pain patient, the pain itself becomes a major barrier to exercise. I encourage you to begin an exercise program, but to consult an interventional physical medicine and rehabilitation specialist if you experience pain that in any way limits your function. The specialist can help diagnose and treat your pain so that it's no longer a barrier to activity or an excuse to remain sedentary.

# CHAPTER 3

# Learn what you should avoid doing each day

Keep moving. Keep striving to improve or at least maintain. If you're not striving, you're coasting — and you can only coast downhill.

Do not sit or stand thoughtlessly.

Strive for the best posture you can achieve. Your mother was right: posture matters! Don't slouch when you sit; don't slouch when you stand.

Avoid compromising your posture when engaging in all activities. Modify your behavior to maintain the best possible posture while participating in day-to-day chores and activities. The most dangerous position for your back is sitting or standing slightly bent forward, such as to wash the dishes or to brush your teeth. These activities are usually what causes your back to "go out" when you're certain you didn't actually "do anything" to injure yourself.

This is why back pain becomes so insidious. For most people, the reasons their back "acts up" are mysterious; it comes on for no apparent reason, unless you understand what we're discussing here. Understanding the mechanism and the physics demystifies the recurrences and allows you to retake control of your back — and your life.

Pay attention to the way you approach simple things like washing the dishes and prepping dinner. We all tend to stand far away from the sink and from the counter when we're working in the kitchen, in order to avoid getting our clothes dirty. This position will create pain in virtually all back pain patients. To avoid this, press your pelvis against the sink or the counter. If you do this properly, you can split your legs, spread your feet, and bend your knees to lower your hands to the level of your work, without ever bending over to wash dishes or cook. (You might look a little strange, but at least you'll be on your way to a pain-free back!)

Don't let wearing clean clothes prevent you from doing this and therefore causing you to injure yourself. Either put on your "chore clothes," or just wear an apron!

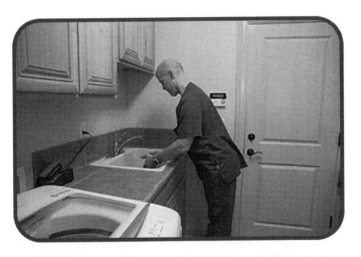

*The wrong way: This puts your discs at risk.*

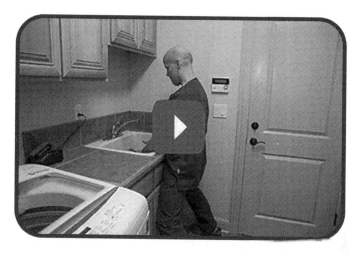

*The right way: This protects your back by keeping it straight. It looks strange, but it sure will help.*

## Running the vacuum

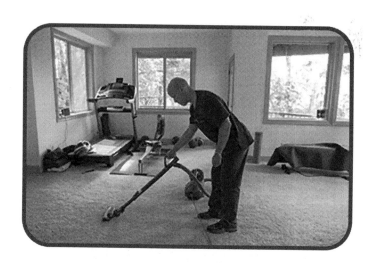

*The wrong way: You're putting your discs at risk by leaning forward.*

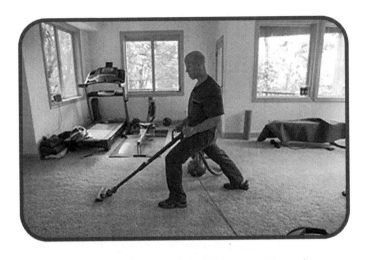

*The right way: Keep your back straight, lengthen the vacuum wand, split your feet, and bend your knees. Looks weird, but it works!*

Use these same principles to change how you do all of your chores and activities.

Take the time to figure out how to do your usual tasks, while thoughtfully and intentionally aligning your spine to neutral.

You can visit whydoihavebackpain.com to view more photos like the ones above and to get further instruction on how to do these various activities without putting your back at risk.

**Don't look to someone else to fix this problem for you. Take ownership.**

Oftentimes you simply won't be aware of the degree to which you're bending forward or to which your back has become asymmetrical as a result of adapting to pain.

Unfortunately, most of us have no idea what to do about back pain or have the habit of looking elsewhere for somebody who can "fix me." No one can fix this problem for you because life, behavior, injury, and pain are constantly driving us into asymmetry. No chiropractor or physical therapist can align your spine for you and keep it there for more than a few hours or days.

But with the right knowledge, information, and understanding, you can fix this problem yourself. The only way to change your spine and reduce the frequency, intensity, and duration of your back pain flare-ups is to change your body from asymmetrical to symmetrical through intentional behavior.

For more chronic or complicated conditions, a highly skilled physical therapist or chiropractor may be necessary to help you better understand the degree to which you've become asymmetrical — not only in the spine, but also in the ligaments, muscles, and tendons that support the spine. This process, though, will only involve manipulating the spine as a tool to help you achieve independence. The evaluation process should really involve a detailed analysis of your body and movement patterns to help you understand where you've become asymmetrical, as well as a customized program to regain your symmetry. But even with this program, you must learn to consciously and actively align your spine into neutral with all activities, at all times.

The first step is simply to know that this is critically important. From there, you have to take ownership of the problem and make it happen.

I encourage you to constantly pay attention to the symmetry of your body. You should look in the mirror frequently (especially when unclothed) to assess for symmetry. Oftentimes you'll find your body has become asymmetrical and that you're leaning to one side or the other — and that you're likely leaning forward without being aware of it.

You'll also probably find that as you try to correct your posture from a left- or right-lean back to the midline, you'll feel like you're leaning in the opposite direction even though you can see in the mirror that you're exactly in the middle. As you look at yourself from the side and attempt to correct a forward lean by standing completely straight, you'll feel pressure in your lower back pushing you forward. If this occurs, it simply means that you've been adapting to this position for long enough that it'll be challenging to correct.

In fact, it might be very painful to correct your posture. But if you fail to follow through, the problem will only get worse. This is the time to be mindful and aware, the time to take action — not to be passive and to give in to the adaptations that have occurred. If this process is simply too painful or time-consuming, it's time to get help from an interventional physical medicine and rehabilitation specialist.

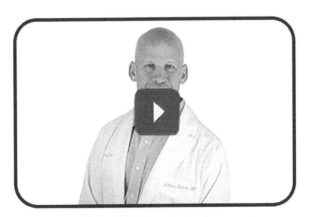

For **Free Video Information**
On This Subject Go To
*whydoihavebackpain.com*

# CHAPTER 4

# Protect your spine

---

Be constantly thoughtful and aware of your spinal alignment at all times. Use your muscles to make yourself tall and straight, both side to side and front to back. Don't let your pain force you to lean forward or to either side.

Teach yourself about protective movement patterns and behaviors. As the images in the last chapter demonstrate, you can always find safer ways to do virtually any task. Always think before you act.

Get used to simply being aware of the position of your spine. The best way to do this is to assess your symmetry whenever you look in the mirror. You can also recruit loved ones to remind you when you're shifting, slouching, or twisting. But be careful: being consistently reminded that you have bad posture can be very irritating. Don't let my advice ruin your marriage! Make an agreement with whomever you ask to help you that they'll attempt to be gentle and funny when reminding you, and constantly tell yourself that you need to be reminded.

Be aware of your body and your strengths and weaknesses. As you go through this process, you'll begin to see where things have become unbalanced. Whether you use a physical therapist or a chiropractor or you decide to investigate through the practice of yoga, the weak links and logjams will become apparent. Your job is to carry that awareness with you all day.

Use your eyes and your brain to thoughtfully align your spine.

Avoid constantly sitting still, no matter how much you focus on your posture. Sedentary behavior will always be your enemy, so get moving! Exercise in a sustainable way as often as possible, but remember that any activity is infinitely better than none at all. Find fun ways to be active, such as gardening or walking in the woods. (Outdoor activities have a host of recognized psychological benefits, so you'll be taking care of your mind while helping your back!)

No one other than yourself (and no path other than your own educated and thoughtful personal efforts) can achieve the goal of proper spinal alignment for you.

There will be times when you can't pinpoint or comprehend the factors preventing you from achieving a symmetrical and properly aligned spine — times when you'll struggle despite your best efforts. At these times, you'll need the help of a physician or structural specialist such as a physical therapist or chiropractor to further understand the issues at hand and what to do about them.

I encourage you to dissect all your activities (especially your primary leisure activities and your occupational activities) to look for things that place you in a shifted, rotated, or forward-flexed position for any length of time. Many of these factors will be modifiable, although some won't be.

Change the things you can change. If you can't change the way you approach any specific activity, you should do your best to change the activity itself.

# CHAPTER 5

# Learn the role of range of motion, strength, and flexibility exercises

If you feel you have a good grip on the posture and behavior issues we've discussed, and if you're not constantly re-injuring your back, you should begin exercising on a regular basis. The goals of your exercise should be to:

1. Improve the quality and quantity of blood flow through aerobic activity. Regular exercise pumps more blood through your tissues, stimulates your body to produce more capillaries, and improves oxygenation of your blood.

2. Improve your joint range of motion. Flexibility training will help you eliminate or reduce the motion restrictions that contribute to chronic spinal shifts and rotations. It will also help you move better through your hips, knees, and ankles so you can get better at the protective movements we discussed.

## Range of motion exercises

As we've discussed, cartilages (joint-lining and disc) don't have blood supplies and are instead nourished by the surrounding bodily fluids. This means that your cartilage essentially breathes; when it's compressed, fluid in the joint and cartilage that's depleted of nutrition and laden with metabolic wastes is squeezed out — and when the pressure is released, fresh fluid that's pH-balanced and loaded with nutrition is drawn in. If your joints aren't moving, they're being starved.

You must move. This is critical to remember, whether you're in the midst of a bad back pain flare-up or you've been feeling fine for some time.

Simply walking is infinitely better than sitting still, but it's also important to go through specifically directed range of motion exercises for all your joints. In my opinion, the best way to achieve this goal is to practice yoga on a regular basis. (Keep in mind that yoga can be dangerous when practiced improperly. This will be addressed in a future book.)

I've emphasized in these pages that you should avoid allowing your back to flex away from the pain — but complete avoidance of flexion can also be counterproductive. What you really want to do is to avoid bending through your lumbar spine while simultaneously bearing the weight of your upper body through your lumbar spine.

Even while you're in pain, it's possible to flex your spine in a non-weight-bearing position. Specifically, you should learn to perform the yoga pose known as cat-cow.

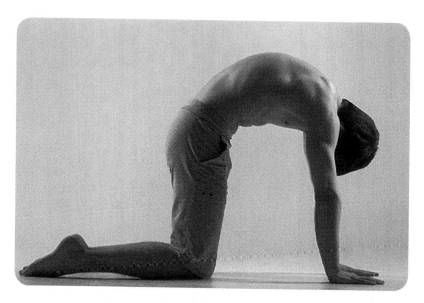

Cat stretch: This allows for a wonderful stretch of the torn part of your disc without putting pressure on the opposite side. You can start doing this even while you're in an acute flare-up.

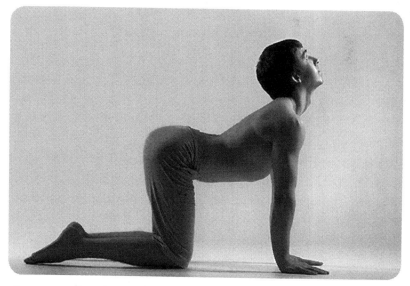

Cow stretch: Always follow cat with cow.

You can safely do cat-cow even during an acute flare-up. Think of these stretches as one; always do cat first, then cow, and repeat multiple times. You can also shift your hips from side to side during the stretch.

I recommend you finish every cat-cow session with one to five minutes of lying prone.

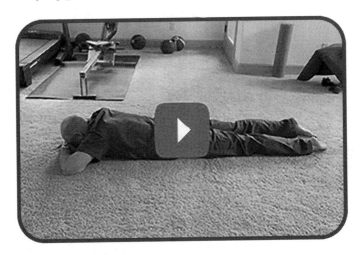

This allows you to relax while preventing you from leaning forward away from your pain. You'll still have to do your best to align your spine and hips in a straight line to achieve the best result.

## Strength and flexibility training

For our purposes here, it's important to note that we're not discussing training for competitive athletes. We're discussing the best methods to achieve the strength and flexibility that will allow you to protect your spine and maintain appropriate posture.

The average person shouldn't follow the "no pain, no gain" paradigm when exercising to improve strength and flexibility.

If you're reading this book, your primary goal should simply be to have less back pain or pain in general. For this reason, you should pursue your exercises with patience and persistence. You should also have in mind a specific reason why you'd like to be stronger and more flexible. In my opinion, the primary goal of these gains should be to improve your ability to master behaviors to protect your spine and your joints. Only when your pain is not limiting your day-to-day function and you're moving freely should you consider the notion of advancing your workouts to include more challenge.

Be cautious with high-intensity interval training and with the current fad of ultra-short workouts. These exercise programs can produce wonderful benefits in a short period of time, but the high intensity involved can place you at risk for injury — so these should be considered advanced workout techniques.

High-intensity workouts will only provide you with exceptional benefits if they're very unpleasant, and most people aren't willing to tolerate this degree of pain. Some people do these high-intensity workouts once or twice and then never do them again because they can't stand to push themselves that hard. The good news? You can still develop a productive exercise habit with workouts that aren't so miserable.

Fitness is a journey that has no destination. Put another way: "With fitness, the journey is the destination."

There will never be a time when you've achieved enough or when the process is over. It's extremely difficult to gain fitness and woefully easy to lose fitness. Once again, remember that your best results will come with patience, persistence, and consistency.

Always remember this mantra on your fitness journey:

Be patient.

Be persistent.

Be consistent.

We're all aging, and I believe it's important to keep this notion in mind: "Life is loss." As we age, every one of us will lose strength, flexibility, balance, agility, reaction time, and aerobic fitness.

If you approach your exercise with the primary goal of *not losing ground as you age*, you'll have the correct mindset. One of the primary difficulties for all people who love to exercise is the challenge of dealing with injury — and one of the primary causes of injury is improper exercise focusing more on intensity rather than form.

I encourage you to reject the "no pain, no gain" philosophy and to focus more on simply challenging yourself. If life isn't challenging, if you're not climbing or at least maintaining, then you're coasting — and you can only coast downhill.

*If you don't feel you have a good grip on what we've discussed, you should visit a physical therapist or chiropractor in your area and ask him or her to help you master the important issues you've learned here. If your state doesn't have open access to physical therapy, try a chiropractor — but please be certain that he or she will focus on helping you master protective behaviors, either directly or through a team. You can also seek out an interventional physical medicine and rehabilitation specialist in your area to better understand the issues at hand and to get a prescription for physical therapy. The prescription for therapy should encourage the therapist to focus on helping you learn how to manage your pain by modifying your behavior, posture, strength, and flexibility.*

# CHAPTER 6

# Learn the role of aerobic exercise

There's ample evidence to demonstrate that people who exercise consistently tend to have healthier joints, healthier spinal discs, and less arthritis in general than people who don't exercise.

Blood flow is critical for healing. Exercise induces a more acute (immediate) blood flow at a higher rate, and consistent exercise expands the vasculature (causes formation of new blood vessels to meet the demands of exercising tissues). Exercise also improves your ability to oxygenate the blood, and well-oxygenated blood allows for better healing.

Given that all the structures we're discussing have either very poor blood supply or none at all, you should be doing anything and everything you can to improve that supply.

During aerobic exercise, your blood supply to all areas increases. Your heart rate and blood pressure go up. You breathe more deeply, which oxygenates your blood more richly — and this, in turn, sends a more robust and vigorous blood supply to all tissues, including the difficult-to-perfuse connective tissues.

It's also clear that those who do exercise have higher oxygenation and better blood flow even at rest than those who don't exercise.

Any activity is better than none, and challenge is good. But to ensure that you'll stay consistent and exercise on a regular basis, you shouldn't challenge yourself at a level that you can't enjoy at least a little.

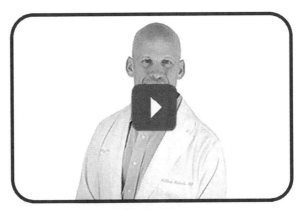

For **Free Video Information**
On This Subject Go To
*whydoihavebackpain.com*

# CHAPTER 7

# Learn the role that rehabilitation services (physical therapy and/or chiropractic) can and should play

I cannot emphasize enough how important the rehabilitation process is. A skilled rehabilitation specialist will be critical to your success if the self-help steps in this book don't do the trick. The fact is that a skilled rehabilitation services provider will be more important to your success in the long run than any orthopedic or spinal interventionalist.

**CASE STUDY #3: Discogenic pain that just needed the appropriate rehabilitation**

WS is a 45-year-old male who presented to the clinic with non-operative, chronic low back pain which he'd experienced for five years.

He was on disability and hadn't worked in years. He'd been through extensive previous physical therapy and pain management (including injections), and he was taking OxyContin with (at best) mild to moderate relief of his pain.

We discussed the fact that he'd already undergone essentially all appropriate injection techniques without significant relief. I advised him that his physical therapy hadn't been properly implemented (as it hadn't focused on the issues we're discussing here) and that seeing a different physical therapist would be his best bet.

As he was severely deconditioned and obese, he was first referred to water therapy before graduating to land-based therapy. The physical therapy focused on spinal stabilization with posture and behavior modification and also on release of adverse neural and dural tension (see page 26).

It took approximately 10 weeks — but on follow-up, he told me that he'd asked his medical pain management doctor to begin tapering him off OxyContin. He had a successful taper, and years later he's doing well. No further injection techniques have been necessary.

Rehabilitation services should focus on:

Learning protective behaviors (structural education, posture, behavior, etc.) so you can stop hurting yourself. Helping you develop strength and flexibility to improve your body's resiliency (resistance to injury). Getting every joint moving normally with home exercise and spinal manipulation/mobilization (manual skills). Spinal manipulation/mobilization should only be used to advance #1 and #2. Improving your blood flow (aerobic exercise process).

Whether this happens through a physical therapist or chiropractor, rehabilitation services should focus initially on assessing the nature of your pain. The provider should observe your motion while asking you to perform a variety of movements to determine which tend to exacerbate your pain and which tend to relieve it. The provider should also observe and palpate your spine for areas of decreased and increased movement as part of the treatment-planning process.

As the vast majority of low back pain originates primarily from your spinal discs, it's important that you never lean away from your pain. The therapist should help you to understand this.

Many rehabilitation providers will instruct you to assume positions that relieve your pain, commonly described as "positions of relief." I've found that this is always a bad idea.

Remember: if your pain is so severe that you can't resist leaning away from it, and if you're not making progress within two weeks despite implementing the methods discussed here, you'll likely need further evaluation by a spine specialist. The specialist will focus on diagnosing any complicating factors (instability, infection, tumor, fracture, etc.) that may require more specific and/or advanced treatment in order for you to advance in therapy. If it turns out that there are no additional complicating pathological factors, then you'll likely need some sort of injection to allow you to make progress in physical therapy.

Adopting postures and positions that acutely relieve your back pain will virtually always make it last longer and make it harder to get rid of in the end. If you can't move into your pain and still maintain normal function, even with the use of medications such as nonsteroidal anti-inflammatory drugs, then it's time to consider an injection to relieve your pain so you don't have to shift away from it.

(A note on nonsteroidal anti-inflammatory drugs: these drugs aren't as safe as once thought. All nonsteroidal anti-inflammatory drugs can cause bleeding from the stomach and kidney-function problems and will double your risk for heart attack and stroke if taken chronically. Furthermore, as inflammation plays an essential role in the healing process from all injuries (whether major or microscopic), theoretically nonsteroidal anti-inflammatory drugs can also significantly decrease your ability to heal and thereby accelerate the degenerative process. For these reasons, nonsteroidal anti-inflammatory drugs should never be taken chronically and should only be used as short-term pain relief while addressing the underlying cause. These factors are magnified substantially in anyone over the age of 50.)

There is a set of safe movements and protective behaviors that can make a major difference in settling your acute flare-ups and preventing future flare-ups. Perhaps the most effective of these is therapeutic prone-lying (lying on your belly while neutralizing your spine from side to side). This position prohibits you from leaning away from your pain, allowing you to rest and relax with a neutral to slightly extended spine. Therapeutic prone-lying should be done frequently for one to five minutes at a time, and its positive effects can be magnified by the use of cat-cow.

For many people, a disc tends to lose motion once it's become injured and painful. This loss of motion makes it very difficult to lean into your pain because the disc isn't moving and is therefore incapable of extending through the injured area. In this case, the palpatory exam and the MRI scan will be helpful in identifying the injured segment. Additionally, if the disc isn't moving, it's also difficult to drive the NP out of the tears and back inside the disc.

## CASE STUDY #4: Lumbar discogenic pain requiring physical therapy to manipulate the L5 and L4 segments as the first step

*PF is a 38-year-old female who presented to my office with lower back pain.*

*She'd been in pain for three years. It started with a non-severe motor vehicle accident resulting in only mild to moderate damage to her car. Her history and physical exam indicated an L5 disc injury — but on physical exam, I couldn't manage to reproduce her pain through active extension of the lumbar spine.*

*Further analysis showed that her L4 and L5 segments weren't moving much at all. When I asked her to bend backwards, all her movement came between L1 and L4.*

*I sent her to physical therapy to work with a skilled manual therapist who could employ manual manipulation skills, McKenzie extension techniques, and my behavior modification protocol to first get her lumbar*

*L4 and L5 segments moving — and then to retrain her posture to reduce her annular tears. She did well without further injection techniques.*

This circumstance requires a skilled provider with manual therapy skills to manipulate your spine, in order to allow the disc to begin to move again. This process can at times be painful. If manipulation of your spine to achieve normal motion is tolerable, the rehabilitation process should proceed.

Once your injured segments are moving, you still need to learn how to consciously and actively align your spine and how to train your behavior to reduce re-injuring the disc and to allow the tear to heal. If this process is too painful, spinal injection techniques can be invaluable in reducing the pain so that manipulation and behavior modification can occur easily, allowing you to make progress.

As the rehabilitation provider works through the passive treatments necessary to help you achieve early relief, he or she should also be focused on helping you understand your pain; how your posture and behavior contribute to your pain; and how your individual strengths and weaknesses and level of flexibility contribute to your asymmetry and the perpetuation of your pain.

As you become more familiar with these factors and as your pain resolves, you should be sent home with specific instructions regarding:

Learning protective behaviors. Modifying your posture and behavior to avoid dangerous positions. Specific exercises for strength and flexibility training to correct your asymmetries and to make you more resilient.

## Neural and Dural tension

These steps will allow you to safely test yourself for chronic neural and dural tension (The Dura Mater is a very tough connective structure that forms the sheath of our entire nervous system extending from the brain through the peripheral nerves) and pain.

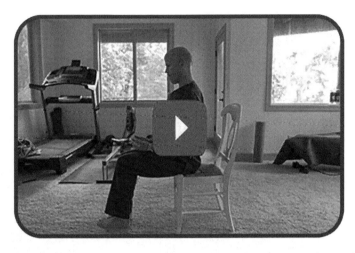

**Step 1:** Sit with good posture, and press your knees together. This will slightly tension your lumbar and sacral nerve roots. Assess for pain reproduction.

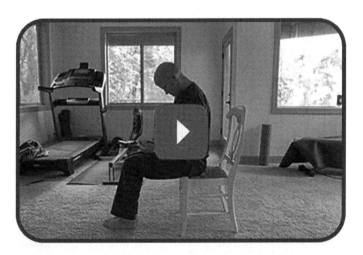

**Step 2:** Tuck your chin gently to your chest. This will begin to elicit tension around your skull, neck, and rib cage. Assess for pain reproduction.

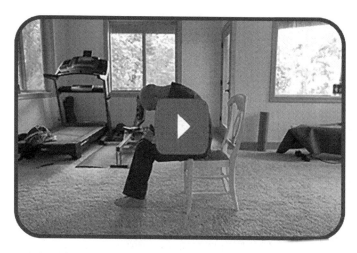

**Step 3:** With your chin tucked, gently slouch as low as your spine will allow. Assess for pain reproduction.

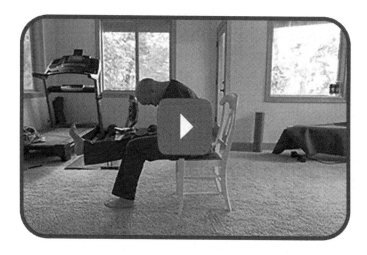

**Step 4:** While slouched as in step 3, straighten one leg and then the other. Assess for pain reproduction.

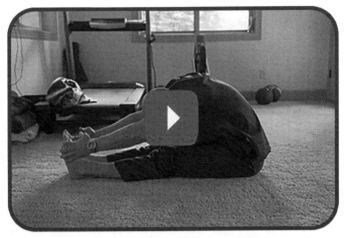

**Step 5:** Sit on the ground with both legs extended in front of you. Intermediate steps may be required to get you from 4 to 5, but this position represents adequate neural flexibility for most people.

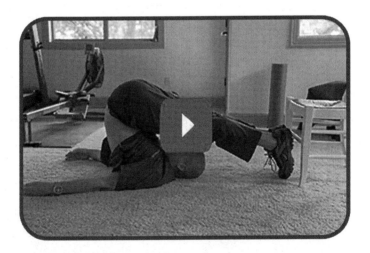

**Step 6:** This is plow pose — the ultimate dural tension stretch. It's advanced, so please visit my page at restorepdx.com for a tutorial on how to achieve it.

Many people with chronic low back pain develop restrictions in the flexibility of the nervous system that can cause more resistant low back pain, as well as secondary painful conditions including sciatica, thoracic back pain, and headaches.

This pathology is called adverse neural and dural tension, which literally means that your nervous system itself (including the actual nerves and the nervous system sheath (the dura mater)) has become pathologically tight as a result of inflammation and adaptation to pain.

Adverse neural tension tends to develop with low back pain, as disc inflammation can easily extend to the sheath of the spinal nerves and as the reduced movement induced by your pain allows the inflamed neural structures to tighten or even to adhere to spinal structures.

Neural and dural tension can be very challenging both to diagnose and to treat and, in fact, shouldn't be treated until your disc has been essentially pain-free for six weeks. This is because the position you must adopt to stretch the nervous system may place an injured disc at risk for further injury if not performed properly. However, if adverse neural and dural tension goes undiagnosed and/or untreated, you likely won't achieve optimal relief and your pain will return sooner rather than later. For some people, adverse neural tension can become the primary cause of chronic disabling pain.

Most providers will teach you to find a position of comfort so you can avoid making your pain worse — which will lead to leaning away from the pain. But by this point, you all know that leaning away from your pain will generally make your pain worse in the long run, even if it feels better at the moment.

Another common mistake is for the rehabilitation provider to start off with strengthening and flexibility exercises, without ever teaching you about protective behaviors. I've found that there's virtually no value in becoming stronger and more flexible if you don't understand why it's important to become stronger and more flexible. If you don't understand that the entire purpose behind increased strength and flexibility is to be able to more effectively correct your posture by adopting protective behaviors, the added strength will not help you.

At the outset of treatment, you may find that you're in such a high degree of pain that the notion of rehabilitation (in the hopes of relief after days or weeks) is simply overwhelming. If your pain has severely disrupted your life, or if you're incapable of concentrating at work, concentrating on your family, or getting through the day without constantly looking for pain medication, then I advise you to consider spinal injection at the beginning of the treatment process, rather than at the end.

Despite the fact that the best injections can only give temporary relief, they can still be critical components in overall treatment if you use the window of opportunity the relief creates to effectively move through the rehabilitation process. I tell my patients that the goal of an early injection is to provide relief so life can go on as normal and you can continue with physical therapy — not to get better, but to learn how to stay better.

But even if an injection produces what appears to be miraculously complete pain relief, you should still go to physical therapy to really understand the underlying issues. This will enable you to learn what you need to know to achieve the most durable response possible from the injection, and it'll give you the critical opportunity to learn protective behaviors.

If your pain is more chronic and indolent (meaning nuisance level rather than life changing) and life is going on fairly normally despite your pain, or if your pain is more of a nuisance than a catastrophic problem, then I encourage you to begin with your rehabilitation provider and to work your way through the process. With appropriate rehabilitation, many people find excellent relief without injection techniques of any kind.

Some people who start with physical therapy find that they're not making significant progress at the end of the first month. At this point, injection techniques can also be a bridge or a lever, allowing you to reach the point where you can truly improve.

It's important to note that the goal of rehabilitation should be not only pain relief but also posture and behavior modification, specifically for restoring symmetry in the spine and symmetry in range of motion. If you don't achieve these goals, you're not truly better — even if you're pain-free.

Consider bringing the below outline to a physical therapist as a point of discussion.

Physical therapy protocol: lumbar discogenic LBP

## Assessment

1. Find and teach position of shift reversal (confirm/deny referring diagnosis/pain provocation pattern).

    a. If discogenic pain diagnosis is confirmed, initiate McKenzie Extension Program.

2. Assess spinal asymmetries: pelvic tilt, lumbosacral lordosis, ilial rotation, lumbar shift, neural/dural, fascial tension.

3. Reassess/confirm/deny referring diagnosis and/or primary pain generator.

4. Assess patient's strength/ability to maintain corrected posture.

5. Assess patient's current/desired level of activity, and adjust strength/proprioceptive (sensing the position of your spine and joints)/balance goals accordingly.

## Mobilization

1. Focus on spine and pelvis/neural structures to reduce above asymmetries.

## Patient training and instruction

1. Intensive training in protective behaviors
2. Strength conditioning of targeted musculature to maintain correct posture at rest and during activity
3. Emphasis on gluteal/pelvic floor/transversus abdominis co-contraction to consciously align spine during all activities
4. Self-mobilization/stretch to achieve or slightly overcorrect asymmetry
5. Continual emphasis on need to actively self-adjust posture to "lean into the pain"
6. Continual cues to the patient to resist the tendency towards antalgic shift, as surrendering to shift will perpetuate pain

## Patient education

1. Emphasize that increased strength and flexibility are of no value if they aren't used to permanently modify posture/behavior/biomechanics.
2. Emphasize behavioral modification to support protective behaviors. Remember: you could easily see excellent resolution of your pain with therapy and/or injections, only to see your pain rapidly return if you haven't been instructed in (and followed through on) protective behavior modification.
3. Teach the importance of maintaining appropriate cardiovascular fitness, generalized strength, and range of motion.
4. Emphasize the recurrent nature of spinal pain and the need to maintain exercise/postural/behavioral modification long-term.

## Home exercise program

1. Emphasize the need to institute and maintain an independent exercise program during physical therapy to allow seamless transition to independent maintenance at conclusion of PT program.

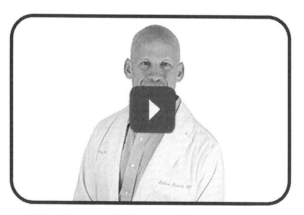

For **Free Video Information**
On This Subject Go To
*whydoihavebackpain.com*

# CHAPTER 8

# Learn the role that spinal injection techniques can and should play

**CASE STUDY #5: Low back pain associated with an L4-L5 fusion, with a resultant combination of L5 discogenic pain and L5-S1 facet joint pain**

JH is an 80-year-old man who presented to me with a chief complaint of lower back pain, ongoing for years after lower back fusion at the level of L4-L5.

He stated that his pain changed after his back surgery but never really got any better. His surgeon had told him that his procedure had been successful and that he had nothing further to offer him.

When I examined the patient, he stood and sat with his low back flexed at approximately 60°. He couldn't stand any straighter than this without very significant pain, and he was walking with a walker set low to accommodate his forward-bent position. He was clearly tender at the bottom of his scar, as well as centrally and approximately two inches to either side of the L5-S1 segment.

I referred him to physical therapy, but he didn't do well. He couldn't tolerate the process of attempting to correct his posture, so he underwent bilateral L5-S1 facet joint injections under x-ray guidance. These injections dramatically relieved his pain, to the point where he came back into my office standing up straight. We discussed moving towards radiofrequency ablation (detailed description of this process in the chapters ahead), but he wasn't interested at that time.

Three months later, he was in my office again, in pain and bent over on his walker. He acknowledged that he didn't go back to physical therapy after the injection, since he was feeling well and didn't think he needed further therapy. At the time of this follow-up visit, he also didn't feel as though he could go back to physical therapy.

For this reason, given that he'd responded well to facet joint injections, I performed L4 and L5 medial branch nerve blocks, which led to radiofrequency ablation of the L4 and L5 bilateral medial branch nerves (to be discussed shortly). The patient did very well with this procedure and came back into my office standing straighter, but not completely straight.

At this point, I convinced him to go back to physical therapy to work on his posture and his behavior. I made it clear that even though the facet joints were hurting him, the L5 disc was under a lot of pressure because of his fusion — and that if he really wanted to feel better for any length of time, he'd have to learn to appropriately modify his posture and his behavior and to perform daily exercises to keep his lumbar spine erect and aligned. He followed through appropriately and did quite well.

One of the most basic principles of my treatment process is that injection techniques should never be used as an isolated or even as a primary treatment.

You should think of these injection techniques as a tool that can: 1) help us be certain that we know what we're treating; and 2) provide rapid significant pain relief in order for you to more effectively participate in physical therapy. In the end, injection techniques are the best way to get better quickly, whereas rehabilitation services are the best way to stay better for the long haul.

You should think about the injection techniques described below in light of the following criteria:

1. Diagnostic value

2. Tools to be used only to advance the therapeutic process to allow patients to better understand the nature of their pain; the nature of their lifestyles and their impact on pain; and the role of posture, behavior, strength, flexibility, nutrition, and physical conditioning on their future with their pain

3. We use spinal injection techniques early in the treatment process to achieve rapid relief when the patient is in high levels of pain and having difficulty living a normal life or when the patient has started physical therapy and simply finds it too painful to tolerate. Injection techniques can rapidly change their ability to tolerate physical therapy.

4. We use injection techniques somewhat later in the process if the current levels of pain are not life-altering — or once the patient has been through four to six weeks of physical therapy and finds that the therapy has been tolerable but hasn't allowed the patient to return to a normal life. At this point, injection techniques can produce enough relief to get past the sticking point in physical therapy and to achieve meaningful relief.

5. When all else has failed, and the appropriate rehabilitation combined with appropriate injections have not produced significant relief, we'll then move on to techniques such as radiofrequency ablation of the medial and lateral branch nerves to relieve pain in a way that'll buy the patient a more durable response, giving them time to continue optimizing their health through better understanding, nutrition, and exercise.

6. The emerging field of regenerative medicine has proven very valuable in getting patients to the point where all the other principles outlined in this book provide the relief necessary for the patient to move on with their lives.

## Epidural steroid injections

### CASE STUDY #6: Lumbar discogenic pain complicated by narrowing of the spinal canal (spinal stenosis) due to degenerative bulges and enlargement of the facet joints

*KN is a 79-year-old woman who presented to my clinic with primarily low back pain.*

*She had a secondary history of painful tightness and fatigue in her thighs that occurred when she'd walk more than 100 feet. Her symptoms clearly suggested discogenic low back pain, which was her primary complaint.*

*Her difficulty walking suggested a condition called neurogenic claudication, which is a result of lumbar spinal stenosis (narrowing of the spinal canal). The narrowing of the spinal canal results from disc bulges along with facet joint enlargement from arthritis. In some cases, it's complicated by a congenitally narrow lumbar spinal canal.*

*Even though the patient had evidence of neurogenic claudication and significant difficulty moving, these weren't her chief complaints. We treated the condition for which she presented: her low back pain, not her symptomatic spinal stenosis.*

*In the past, she'd undergone partially successful radiofrequency ablation of the lumbar medial branch nerve to control facet joint pain. Her physical exam was very clearly positive for antalgic shift forward and slightly to the right to control her primarily left-sided lower back pain. I sent her to physical therapy to work on her posture.*

*Conventional medical wisdom suggests that the lumbar spine shouldn't be extended when there's significant evidence of neurogenic claudication related to lumbar spinal stenosis. Given that the patient's primary complaint was lower back pain (which I attributed to her disc bulging at L4 and L5), I felt it was valuable to treat her primary condition despite the potential contraindication to extension-based treatment. (A common notion amongst medical practitioners is that extending the spine narrows the canal and shouldn't be suggested to persons with spinal stenosis.)*

*The patient underwent a single bilateral L4 transforaminal epidural steroid injection and saw significant relief of her pain. This allowed her to work effectively in physical therapy to correct her posture so that, when I next saw her, she was standing straight and feeling dramatically better. She's done well ever since and continues to work daily on her posture and her behavioral biomechanics.*

It's interesting that, despite the fact that the lumbar disc in and of itself is the most common cause (either directly or indirectly) of lower back pain, our interventional procedures have very little impact directly on the disc. The most commonly used interventional procedures are more effective for treating secondary conditions like facet joint pain, sacroiliac joint pain, hip joint pain, and myofascial trigger points.

But that's not to say that injection techniques aren't valuable for relieving discogenic pain and advancing therapy.

Epidural steroid injections delivered can be delivered in three distinct ways, (interlaminar, transforaminal or caudal) each has it's own peculiar risks and advantages which should be addressed by your interventionalist. Epidural steroid injections can definitely be helpful. The key precaution is to never use these injection techniques as the only intervention. They do nothing about the underlying cause of the situation and can only produce a temporary response if not used as part of a comprehensive spinal rehabilitation program.

After virtually every successful epidural cortisone injection for back and leg pain, my patients ask how long the relief will last. The textbooks will tell you that the duration of relief from these injections is roughly three months; however, if you rely on the injection to produce durable relief, you'll likely be very disappointed.

From what I can tell, the epidural cortisone produces relief quickly — but the medication rapidly leaves your system as well. I believe that when you respond to injection and follow up in two weeks thinking that the shot is "still working," the shot's effects have lapsed and you're only better because you haven't re-injured the area.

By the two-week mark, the medications are effectively gone from the injection site even though you continue to feel substantially improved. For this reason, it seems clear that when your symptoms eventually recur, the flare-up won't be due to a failure of the durability of the injection but rather because of a new injury to the same area. As such, even after a successful injection, it's critically important to follow through with physical therapy in order to achieve a long-term response.

Why would we expect an epidural cortisone injection to help with discogenic pain?

1. We know that most painful injuries to the lumbar disc are in the posterior third of the AF, which sits in the epidural space of the spine. We know that when the NP contacts any part of the spine that's not genetically designed to contain it (including the nerve roots), it will cause significant inflammation and subsequently back pain and/or sciatica. This suggests that we can relieve inflammation and, thus, the pain if we put cortisone directly on these inflamed structures.

2. When the NP has invaded a tear of the disc, the substance of the AF becomes so swollen that it effectively traps the invading NP within the tear. This can prevent that portion of the NP from retreating back into its pocket. It's then logical that reducing inflammation across the back front of the AF can facilitate extension-based therapy, as well as posture and behavior modification.

## Intradiscal injections

Intradiscal injections are controversial. The risks are low, but the potential exists for the needle puncture in the annulus to create an injury that can cause pain. If the disc becomes infected with injection, surgery is often necessary. As a result, these injections are left for late-stage intervention.

Most intradiscal injections are performed diagnostically. Up until about 10 to 15 years ago, a procedure called provocation diagnostic discography was very commonly used as a tool to diagnose which level discs in the lumbar spine were painful. Provocation discography involved pressurizing the inside of the disc to reproduce pain for diagnostic purposes. Provocation discography has fallen out of favor.

Diagnosing lumbar disc pain and specifying which levels are painful is still valuable, particularly when considering intradiscal regenerative treatments. For this purpose, we tend to use local anesthetic injections of the disc. In this intradiscal injection, a small amount of a concentrated local anesthetic is injected into the center of the disc under low pressure. This local anesthetic will then spread into the AF and provide an anesthetic effect. As with other spinal injections, we're looking for a negative response — meaning we're looking for pain relief, not pain reproduction.

Spinal injection techniques can provide excellent relief for low back and associated leg pain. Fortunately, many patients understand that this relief is temporary, so they prefer not to use spinal injection techniques as "they're only a Band-Aid" and they don't want to become dependent on injections to relieve their pain.

In our hands, spinal injection techniques are a valuable tool and nothing more. These techniques are used for diagnosis and to advance the treatment process. Spinal injection techniques should never be the only treatment. When used as the primary treatment, spinal injection techniques are doomed to failure.

## Injection techniques to treat the lumbar facet joints

## CASE STUDY #7: Discogenic pain complicated by an underlying facet joint problem

*EY is a 30-year-old male who's had chronic low back pain for the last 12 years.*

*Before coming to see me, he'd been to multiple medical centers, including locations that are widely considered to be world leaders in medical care.. When he came to me, he said he'd been treated for his degenerative L5 disc with physical therapy and epidural steroid injections. On further questioning, he revealed that the physical therapy never included behavior modification or a clear focus on posture. It was obvious to me that his pain was, in fact, discogenic and that the epidural cortisone injection would likely be at least temporarily effective for his condition — but these had already been performed at other facilities.*

*It was also clear that he hadn't had the appropriate physical therapy. For this reason, I sent him to physical therapy first. After two weeks, he came back saying that the physical therapy was causing his pain to flare up. When I reviewed his MRI scan, I saw that he did have some inflammation and degeneration of the facet joints.*

*I realized I had to come up with a different treatment plan, since he'd already undergone epidural cortisone injections (which hadn't made a big difference) and as physical therapy was causing pain. We discussed facet joint injections, even though facet joint pain in a 30-year-old is relatively uncommon.*

*Nevertheless, these injections provided him with very good relief for a short period. This then led to medial branch nerve blocks and eventually to radiofrequency ablation of the medial branch nerves — which finally provided him with excellent relief.*

*This relief allowed him to participate in physical therapy to modify his posture and his behavior. From that point forward, his condition improved considerably.*

Although back pain is virtually always either directly or indirectly related to the lumbar disc, other structures can contribute significantly to pain and that often must be treated through injection techniques.

The most common of these structures are the lumbar facet joints and the sacroiliac joint. Other less commonly involved structures are the hip joints and the other ligaments around the pelvis.

As the human body ages and lumbar disc injuries lead to both symmetrical and non-symmetrical collapse, degeneration, and antalgic adaptation in posture and behavior, the body will become progressively more asymmetric. This leads to degeneration of secondary structures that may become painful. The most common of these are the lumbar facet joints and sacroiliac joints.

There are times when the structures will become so painful that they must be diagnosed and treated separately, and there are times when the lumbar facet joints become arthritic and painful, contributing to the patient's inability to properly align his or her spine into a neutral position. Once the facet joints are significantly painful, it becomes all but impossible to biomechanically treat the lumbar disc.

When a patient adapts to lumbar pain through lumbar shifts and rotations, the uneven torque to the sacroiliac joints that results can produce significant pain that prevents working toward symmetry and the proper biomechanical treatment of the lumbar disc. Proper injection techniques can be a critical tool in diagnosing and treating sacroiliac joint pain.

As a basic rule, spinal injections must be performed very accurately and with appropriate image guidance — which at this time, in all cases for the spine, means the use of fluoroscopy (an imaging technique that allows you to see bony structures inside the body in real-time) to specifically and selectively anesthetize certain structures.

The theory is that, if your right-side L4-L5 and L5-S1 facet joints are a major source of your pain, I can place a needle in these joints and make them completely numb — during which time your pain will be gone. For this reason, injection should be done very specifically and very selectively, and you should always be provided with a pain diary.

The pain diary should specifically show your pain level immediately before the procedure, your pain level when your pain is at its worst, and the activity you're doing when the pain rises to its worst. Your pain number should then be recorded immediately after the injection, then every 15 minutes for one hour, then once an hour for eight hours. You should be instructed to be thoughtfully active after the injection — to go back to your daily activities thinking very carefully about whether or not we've resolved your pain. If you feel somewhat better, you should then do things that would usually make your pain worse to determine whether we've injected the proper spot.

If the injection provided dramatic pain relief, you've achieved the diagnosis. The initial injection will usually contain a very small amount of corticosteroid in order to also relieve inflammation. This component of the injection also provides diagnosis, since it permits us to determine the specific cause of your pain. The point is that injected corticosteroids are so powerfully anti-inflammatory that, if you don't achieve sustained relief, it means the injected structure is mechanically painful rather than inflamed. In other words, if you do achieve significant relief, then the structure is significantly inflamed; if you don't achieve immediate relief, the structure wasn't a specific cause of your pain.

If you don't achieve relief on the day of the injection but your pain begins to significantly settle down a day or two later, you have inflammation — but it's not near the injected structure. This usually means that the search for the specific cause of your pain should continue until an injection achieves immediate and dramatic relief.

Typical outcomes from facet joint injections include:

1. You achieve no relief of any kind.

   a. This means the facet joints are not causing your pain, and so the search for the source of your pain should continue.

2.  Your pain is completely or dramatically relieved for several hours or a couple of days, but it then returns.

    a.  This means the facet joints are causing your pain. But the lack of durable relief means the joints aren't inflamed, so further cortisone injections won't be valuable. You'll likely move on to radiofrequency ablation.

3.  Your pain is completely and immediately relieved, and the relief is ongoing.

    a.  This means that the facet joints are causing your pain and that they were inflamed. You should now be progressing in physical therapy to adopt protective behaviors and to modify your posture.

4.  You achieve no immediate relief, but lasting relief starts days after the injection.

    a.  This means you have inflammatory pain near the facet joints but the joints injected aren't the primary cause of your pain. If the relief is adequate, you should move on with physical therapy to modify your posture and behavior.

Oftentimes, a single injection will provide such significant relief that physical therapy which had been stalled or simply too painful to tolerate will suddenly progress to the point of pain resolution.

If a single injection provides this result and you feel as though you're completely pain-free, please don't be tempted to abandon therapy until you've achieved complete symmetry of range of motion and posture through the painful structure, and you're certain that you can and will continue with protective behaviors.

In more complex cases, particularly when it comes to injections of the facet joints or the sacroiliac joint, you might have immediate and complete relief of pain for several hours after the injection that doesn't continue for any significant length of time. As stated above, this would mean the injected structure is in fact a major contributor to your pain but that it's not inflamed. Under this circumstance, once physical therapy has become overly painful or has stalled completely, moving on to radiofrequency ablation of the appropriate sensory nerves can provide meaningful, long-lasting relief — so that, once again, you can achieve the major goals of therapy: mastering protective behaviors, restoring symmetrical posture, and normal range of motion.

Lumbar facet joint injections can only be done through fluoroscopy (a moving x-ray), which allows you to actually see the joints and have a chance of placing medication inside the joint. These injections are generally done with a combination of local anesthetic and injectable cortisone.

These injections provide a few potential benefits.

The first goal of facet joint injections is diagnostic. We follow the theory that a selected potential generator (where your pain is coming from) will stop causing pain immediately or in very short order when it's injected with a chemical to make it temporarily numb. For this reason, all patients receiving a facet joint injection are advised to assess their pain immediately before the injection and to number it in relation to its very worst in the last days to weeks (with 1 being the lowest level and 10 the highest).

Pain Diary

Matthew G. Michaels, MD

| Patient Name | DOB |
|---|---|
| Procedure Date | Procedure End Time |
| Procedure Description | |

| | 0 | Pain Free. |
|---|---|---|
| Tolerable | 1 | I can live with this pain level just fine |
| | 2 | |
| | 3 | I do NOT need medical help for this level of pain |
| | 4 | I can still do what I want/need to do without struggle<br>Over the counter pain remedies are effective |
| Barely Tolerable | 5 | I want medical/professional help with this pain.<br>Daily activities are a struggle |
| | 6 | |
| | 7 | I need to get some help from a doctor.<br>I can't enjoy fun time because of the pain<br>Pain makes it difficult to concentrate, interferes with sleep. |
| Not Tolerable | 8 | Physical activity severely limited. You can read and converse only with effort.<br><br>Nausea and dizziness set in as factors of pain. |
| | 9 | Unable to speak. Need to go to the Emergency Room for help NOW. |
| | 10 | Need an AMBULANCE to go to the Emergency room for help. Pain makes you pass out. |

**PRE-PROCEDURE BASELINE PAIN LEVEL**

**Pain Rating**  0 ------- 1 ------- 2 ------- 3 ------- 4 ------- 5 ------- 6 ------- 7 ------- 8 ------- 9 ------- 10

No Pain         Tolerable         Not Tolerable         Worst Possible Pain

| Time after Procedure | Average Pain-Scale Rating After Your Procedure |
|---|---|
| 1 minute | 0 ——— 1 ——— 2 ——— 3 ——— 4 ——— 5 ——— 6 ——— 7 ——— 8 ——— 9 ——— 10 |
| 15 minutes | 0 ——— 1 ——— 2 ——— 3 ——— 4 ——— 5 ——— 6 ——— 7 ——— 8 ——— 9 ——— 10 |
| 30 minutes | 0 ——— 1 ——— 2 ——— 3 ——— 4 ——— 5 ——— 6 ——— 7 ——— 8 ——— 9 ——— 10 |
| 45 minutes | 0 ——— 1 ——— 2 ——— 3 ——— 4 ——— 5 ——— 6 ——— 7 ——— 8 ——— 9 ——— 10 |
| 1 hour | 0 ——— 1 ——— 2 ——— 3 ——— 4 ——— 5 ——— 6 ——— 7 ——— 8 ——— 9 ——— 10 |
| 2 hours | 0 ——— 1 ——— 2 ——— 3 ——— 4 ——— 5 ——— 6 ——— 7 ——— 8 ——— 9 ——— 10 |
| 3 hours | 0 ——— 1 ——— 2 ——— 3 ——— 4 ——— 5 ——— 6 ——— 7 ——— 8 ——— 9 ——— 10 |
| 4 hours | 0 ——— 1 ——— 2 ——— 3 ——— 4 ——— 5 ——— 6 ——— 7 ——— 8 ——— 9 ——— 10 |
| 5 hours | 0 ——— 1 ——— 2 ——— 3 ——— 4 ——— 5 ——— 6 ——— 7 ——— 8 ——— 9 ——— 10 |
| 6 hours | 0 ——— 1 ——— 2 ——— 3 ——— 4 ——— 5 ——— 6 ——— 7 ——— 8 ——— 9 ——— 10 |
| 7 hours | 0 ——— 1 ——— 2 ——— 3 ——— 4 ——— 5 ——— 6 ——— 7 ——— 8 ——— 9 ——— 10 |
| 8 hours | 0 ——— 1 ——— 2 ——— 3 ——— 4 ——— 5 ——— 6 ——— 7 ——— 8 ——— 9 ——— 10 |
| 1 day | 0 ——— 1 ——— 2 ——— 3 ——— 4 ——— 5 ——— 6 ——— 7 ——— 8 ——— 9 ——— 10 |
| 2 days | 0 ——— 1 ——— 2 ——— 3 ——— 4 ——— 5 ——— 6 ——— 7 ——— 8 ——— 9 ——— 10 |
| 3 days | 0 ——— 1 ——— 2 ——— 3 ——— 4 ——— 5 ——— 6 ——— 7 ——— 8 ——— 9 ——— 10 |
| 4 days | 0 ——— 1 ——— 2 ——— 3 ——— 4 ——— 5 ——— 6 ——— 7 ——— 8 ——— 9 ——— 10 |
| 5 days | 0 ——— 1 ——— 2 ——— 3 ——— 4 ——— 5 ——— 6 ——— 7 ——— 8 ——— 9 ——— 10 |
| 6 days | 0 ——— 1 ——— 2 ——— 3 ——— 4 ——— 5 ——— 6 ——— 7 ——— 8 ——— 9 ——— 10 |
| 7 days | 0 ——— 1 ——— 2 ——— 3 ——— 4 ——— 5 ——— 6 ——— 7 ——— 8 ——— 9 ——— 10 |
| 8 days | 0 ——— 1 ——— 2 ——— 3 ——— 4 ——— 5 ——— 6 ——— 7 ——— 8 ——— 9 ——— 10 |
| 9 days | 0 ——— 1 ——— 2 ——— 3 ——— 4 ——— 5 ——— 6 ——— 7 ——— 8 ——— 9 ——— 10 |
| 10 days | 0 ——— 1 ——— 2 ——— 3 ——— 4 ——— 5 ——— 6 ——— 7 ——— 8 ——— 9 ——— 10 |
| 11 days | 0 ——— 1 ——— 2 ——— 3 ——— 4 ——— 5 ——— 6 ——— 7 ——— 8 ——— 9 ——— 10 |
| 12 days | 0 ——— 1 ——— 2 ——— 3 ——— 4 ——— 5 ——— 6 ——— 7 ——— 8 ——— 9 ——— 10 |
| 13 days | 0 ——— 1 ——— 2 ——— 3 ——— 4 ——— 5 ——— 6 ——— 7 ——— 8 ——— 9 ——— 10 |
| 14 days | 0 ——— 1 ——— 2 ——— 3 ——— 4 ——— 5 ——— 6 ——— 7 ——— 8 ——— 9 ——— 10 |

**PLEASE BRING THIS FORM WITH YOU**
**TO YOUR FOLLOW-UP APPOINTMENT OR FAX TO (  )  -**

They're then asked to assess their pain immediately after the injection (disregarding the residual pain they may have from the needle or the injection itself) and then to continue to assess their pain every 15 minutes for the next hour. If, at the end of that hour, they're convinced the pain has significantly lessened, they're then asked to go out and do the activities they'd previously noted had increased pain. If they find they simply cannot reproduce their pain, or that the pain is dramatically reduced (enough to significantly improve function) from the local anesthetic effect of the injection, we then have a diagnosis that the facet joints are causing the patient's pain.

Follow-up after these injections is typically in a week.

The low-dose cortisone in the injection also plays a diagnostic role. Injectable corticosteroids are extremely powerful anti-inflammatory medications. For this reason, it's thought that if the patient achieves significantly ongoing relief for more than a few hours (extending to a couple of days) after a facet joint injection, it's likely the facet joints were both painful and inflamed.

If the patient notes that he or she is seeing significant ongoing relief from facet joint injection at the one-week mark, they're sent to physical therapy to facilitate mastery of protective behaviors, posture and behavior modification, and therapeutic exercise (which includes strength and flexibility training to facilitate the most durable possible response to the cortisone injected into the joint).

## Lumbar medial branch nerve blocks

If the patient achieves very significant relief for the first several hours after the facet joint injection, but finds the pain returning to nearly its original level in a few short hours or days after the injection, we then assume that: 1) the joint is painful but not inflamed as it didn't respond to steroid; and 2) further steroid injections would be counterproductive and more likely to lead to significant side effects.

At this point, we generally move on to medial branch nerve blocks.

The medial branch nerves are very small nerves roughly half an inch long and about the thickness of two human hairs twisted together. These nerves do very little other than supply innervation to the facet joints and a small muscle (called the multifidus) that sits between the segments of the spine.

The medial branch nerves always sit in a very specific and reliable area. X-ray guidance is used to place fine needles directly onto the spot where we know the medial branch nerves live. At this point, roughly two drops of x-ray contrast dye are injected to confirm the medication is going into the right spot and will stay there, rather than being washed away by a vein that might sit in the same area.

When we're sure we're in the right spot and that the medication will stay where we want it, we inject roughly two drops of a powerful local anesthetic (in our clinic, 0.5% ropivacaine). Once again, the patient is asked to comment on the pain immediately before and immediately after the injection and to perform those usually painful activities after the injection. If, the patient experiences significant but short-duration pain relief, we then move on to radiofrequency ablation of the medial branch nerves.

## Radiofrequency ablation of the medial branch nerves

Radiofrequency ablation is also known as the hot needle treatment or "burning the nerves."

The nerves we're targeting aren't involved in any way in skin sensation or muscular control in your pelvis or legs. These nerves control sensation in the facet joints and the bones of the posterior (rear-facing) elements, and supply sensation to the small muscle mentioned above (the multifidus).

This procedure uses localized, specifically directed heat to produce injure a very small area. This injury to the medial branch nerve must heal before the nerve can once again send pain signals to the brain. This healing process takes anywhere from six to 12 months.

This injury doesn't kill the medial branch nerves — which is both good and bad: It's good that the nerve isn't dead, as you can be assured that the procedure won't permanently change anything, but it's bad that it doesn't kill the nerve because, if the procedure works, we know the relief won't be permanent. The nerve will heal and the pain might come back.

However, if the procedure's done properly and actually works, we'll then send you to physical therapy so that, during the pain-free phase, you can work on your posture, behavior, strength, flexibility, and overall conditioning. This allows us to create the possibility that your pain won't return when the nerve heals, as the underlying problem has changed with your improved condition.

## Radiofrequency ablation technique

To most people, this particular intervention sounds brutal. The notion of burning nerves in the lower back is disturbing but, when performed properly, it can be nearly pain-free and performed with you wide-awake — meaning entirely without sedation.

The procedure is typically done on one side and usually targets no more than three nerves at a time. The most common levels for ablation are the lumbar three, four, and five medial branch nerves.

The procedure starts with cleaning (sterilizing) that area of your skin and isolating the area with sterile drapes. We then use the fluoroscope to determine the appropriate trajectory for optimally placing the needles. We then anesthetize your skin using a very fine 27-gauge needle.

Then the ablation needle (typically an 18-gauge needle that's insulated for all but the last 10mm, to allow only the uninsulated portion to transmit heat to the area around it) is inserted through the anesthetized skin and placed on the bone at the level of the nerve to be ablated. At this point, about 1cc of 1% lidocaine (a very short-lived but rapid-acting local anesthetic) is injected to numb the nerves in the entire area.

The same procedure is then repeated for the remaining two levels.

In this front view, we're very careful not to place the needles too deep. We obtain a side view and advance the needle to the appropriate depth.

Inside the needle is a probe, which is attached to a machine that heats the tip of the needle and the surrounding area. The needle is heated to 80°C for 90 seconds. The position of the needle tip may then be adjusted once or twice for an additional one or two burn spots, depending on the anatomy and the circumstances.

In most cases, the patient barely feels anything. He or she will usually have a Band-Aid on the skin at each needle puncture, but will be allowed to go home within minutes after the procedure is done with no specific precautions. We'll typically follow up with our patients at the two-week mark.

## Potential failure of lumbar radiofrequency ablation technique

The clinical research and our experience suggest that about 70% of all patients have an immediate positive response, with relief lasting anywhere from six months to a year.

Of the 30% that don't have an immediate positive response, most show clear relief at the level of the burn spot but still have pain below it (usually roughly at the bottom of the sacroiliac joint or in the area of the S4 posterior nerve root).

My experience is that nearly all these patients will respond that day to a single injection of lidocaine at the point of maximal tenderness in the tailbone area. After this injection, virtually all walk out of the office pain-free.

Roughly half those patients will have a long-lasting response and not need any further treatment until the ablation wears off in roughly six months to a year. The remaining half will have temporary relief and will come back to the office in one week with ongoing pain in the tailbone area. These patients generally have sacroiliac joint pain, which will respond beautifully to treatment as delineated below.

## Injection techniques to treat sacroiliac joint pain

### CASE STUDY #8: Low back pain associated with sacroiliac joint pain after extensive lumbar fusion from L3 through the sacrum

*KN is a 53-year-old female who, four years previously, underwent lumbar fusion for low back and leg pain.*

*She stated that the surgery had been both successful and unsuccessful. Certain components of her pain had gotten better, and others had gotten worse. Since that time, she'd been on and off narcotics and had been to extensive physical therapy and interventional pain management without significant relief.*

*She was on narcotics when she visited me and expressed a desire to get off them. Her physical exam showed clear evidence of tenderness of the sacroiliac joints. This had been treated in the past with injection but hadn't been addressed in physical therapy with posture and behavior management. The injections had provided temporary relief lasting no more than a couple of weeks at most.*

*Due to her high levels of pain, I decided we should proceed through lateral branch nerve block and then possibly onto lateral branch radiofrequency ablation if the lateral branch nerve blocks were successful. This process went smoothly, and she achieved 90% pain relief through sacral lateral branch nerve radiofrequency ablation.*

*She then went to physical therapy, where multiple musculoskeletal issues were addressed — including tightness of her hip flexor muscles and weakness of her gluteal muscles. She was retrained regarding movement, behavior, and posture and given a home-exercise program.*

*At the eight-week mark, her symptoms were completely resolved, and she'd begun tapering off her narcotics with her primary care doctor.*

## CASE STUDY #9: Lumbar discogenic and sciatic nerve pain complicated by sacroiliac joint pain and narrowing of the L5 foramen as a result of a prolonged lumbar shift

*HR is a 60-year-old male who presented to my office with a primary complaint of left-leg numbness when standing.*

*He didn't complain of low back pain on presentation — but on observing his stance and his gait, it became obvious that he was shifted to the left through his lumbar spine and that he was bearing virtually all of his bodyweight on his left leg.*

*When I asked him to shift his weight toward the right, he complained of fairly intense right-sided low back pain. The fact is that the right-sided pain was the result of an old injury that he'd adapted to by shifting his body weight toward the left. This had resolved the low back pain but had caused a whole new problem: narrowing of his nerve root openings on the left side as a result of shifting his weight to that side.*

*In this case, physical therapy focused on correcting the lumbar shift into his right-sided lower back pain. It took a little bit of persuasion to help the patient understand that in order for his left leg symptoms to resolve, he'd have to work through his right-sided low back pain.*

*He also required spinal injections to treat his right sacroiliac joint pain and a consequent ablation of the right L5, S1, S2, S3, and S4 lateral branch nerves. This dramatically reduced his right-sided low back and buttock pain, and he then managed to change his posture — shifting his weight to an equal stance bilaterally, which allowed his left-leg numbness to dissipate.*

The approach here is the same as for facet joint injections. We use a fluoroscope to place the needle in the sacroiliac joint and then inject, making sure the medication goes where we want it. We then inject the joint with a combination of local anesthetic, corticosteroid, and dextrose to anesthetize and decrease inflammation in the joint.

These are typical outcomes from sacroiliac joint injections:

1.  You achieve no relief of any kind.

    a.  This means the sacroiliac joints aren't causing your pain and the search for the source should continue.

2.  Your pain is completely or dramatically relieved for several hours or a couple of days, but it then returns.

    a.  This means the sacroiliac joints are causing your pain — but the lack of durable relief means the joints aren't inflamed, so further cortisone injections won't be valuable. You'll likely move on to radiofrequency ablation.

3.  Your pain is completely and immediately relieved, and the relief is ongoing.

    a.  This means the sacroiliac joints were inflamed and causing your pain. You should now progress in physical therapy to modify your posture and behavior.

4.  You achieve no immediate relief, but lasting relief starts days after the injection.

    a.  This means you have inflammatory pain near the sacroiliac joints but that the injected joints aren't the primary cause of your pain. If the relief is adequate, you should move on with physical therapy to modify your posture and behavior.

## Lateral branch nerve blocks

Lateral branch nerve blocks are a diagnostic test designed to determine whether radiofrequency ablation of the lateral branch nerves might be useful in managing your pain.

The sacral lateral branch nerves are sensory only and don't control anything other than sensation from the sacroiliac joint and the ligament behind the joint. Most of the research performed on sacral lateral branch nerve ablation has focused on the first, second, and third lateral branch nerves. The studies generally result in a roughly 60% response rate to ablation of those nerves.

My experience with local treatment of the S4 level leads me to believe that ablation of the fourth sacral lateral branch nerve is critical to treatment of sacroiliac joint pain with radiofrequency ablation. I don't have evidence to prove this is true, but my experience and patient success have shown me a near-80% response rate for lumbosacral lateral branch ablation from L4 through S4. I believe this is due to treatment of the S4 level.

As noted above, I target five separate nerves with the potential or proven ability to supply sensation to the sacroiliac joint. For this procedure, five separate 25-gauge spinal needles are simultaneously placed, under x-ray guidance, at the margin of the rear-facing nerve opening closest to the joint.

As in the lumbar medial nerve branch block, a small amount of contrast dye is injected to ensure the medication will flow where we want it to. Then, we inject about half a cc of a long-acting, concentrated local anesthetic to anesthetize the nerves.

The patient is then asked to return home and assess the pain. If the patient thinks it's better, we ask him or her to perform the activities that would normally exacerbate the pain to be certain the patient has achieved solid 75% relief. Significant relief from lateral branch nerves is generally quite temporary and will usually lead to radiofrequency ablation.

## Sacral lateral branch nerve ablation technique

As with the lumbar medial branch nerve ablation technique, the sacral lateral branch nerve ablation technique sounds brutal — but it's actually relatively painless.

The key difference between ablation of the lateral branch nerves of the sacrum and the medial branch nerves of the lumbar spine is that the lateral branch nerves of the sacrum are less reliably in the exact same spot on every person.

The variability of positioning requires the performance of a more thorough ablation. This is done through the use of what's called parallel lesioning. In the conventional technique used for cervical and lumbar medial branch nerve ablation, the electricity used to degenerate the nerve travels between the tip of the needle and a grounding pad (a 4-inch square pad stuck to the skin that acts as a point of exit for the electrical current that flows from the tip of the needle). This concentrates all the heat around the tip of the needle in roughly the shape of a cotton swab tip.

In parallel lesioning, the ground pad is taken out of the circuit, and the electricity runs between two needles. The heat then forms a complex shape between the two needles, so long as they're no more than roughly one centimeter apart.

We place the needles in such a way that each one uses only one skin-entry point and is adjusted at depth for each subsequent lesion. The four needles are placed at the top of the sacrum, roughly one centimeter apart to lesion the L5, S1, and S2 lateral branch nerves.

The parallel component of the lesion is run between needles one and two and then between needles three and four. All four needles are then repositioned toward the bottom of the sacrum by roughly one to one-and-a-half centimeters. An additional parallel lesion is created at this point. The needles are then moved toward the bottom of the sacrum by roughly another one to one-and-a-half centimeters. Depending on the patient's size, the same process is repeated another one or two times to achieve ablation from L5 through S4.

Most people experience immediate relief with little discomfort afterward. Some people experience bruising, and some discomfort from it, after the procedure.

If a patient goes through one of these interventional procedures and obtains significant relief, it's still not a good idea to neglect further therapy and treatment. At this point, it's critical to continue at home with ongoing cognitive and active alignment of the spine during all activities, in order to achieve optimal posture and movement in day-to-day life.

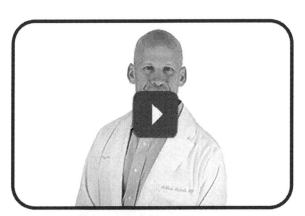

For **Free Video Information**
On This Subject Go To
*whydoihavebackpain.com*

# CHAPTER 9

# Learn the role that surgical intervention can and should play

Certain conditions are strictly surgical. In other words: when you need a good surgeon, you really need a good surgeon.

In clinical practice, my goal is to do my best to treat appropriate conditions non-surgically, while making it clear when non-surgical intervention isn't the right option. A non-surgical spinal specialist should not give you the impression that they are trying to dissuade you from having surgery, but rather to make it clear that you often have other options.

It's important to understand that the vast majority of back surgery is elective. There are very few reasons why patients actually *need* surgery on their spines.

Pain is not one of those reasons. Surgery for a degenerative painful spine is an elective surgery.

The list of reasons why spinal surgery should be performed include:

1. Frank instability of the spine due to trauma, degeneration, various types of listhesis (vertebrae sliding off each other due to arthritis or stress fracture), infection, or tumor. Frank instability means that specific segments of your spine are moving relative to each other to such a degree that they place your spinal nerves and/or spinal cord at risk for injury from compression related to the excessive movement. There is no appropriate solution to this problem other than surgical fusion of the spinal segments that have become unstable.

2. Compression of the spinal nerves causing progressive loss of strength. In this circumstance, the surgery is performed to prevent further loss of strength — because, once significant weakness due to nerve damage has occurred, it's unlikely that strength will return any time soon (if at all). As such, simple static numbness or static weakness doesn't make spinal surgery medically necessary.

3. Spinal infection and tumors. These must often be treated surgically even if they haven't caused instability.

Spinal surgery doesn't guarantee a positive outcome. Many spinal surgeries, including fusions and decompressions, result in no significant improvement or even worsening of pain.

It's also important to note that in many of the cases that do get significant benefit from surgery, late complications often occur that lead to accelerated pathology in structures adjacent to the operated spinal segments. Nevertheless, once surgery has been performed, there are options to treat any negative outcome.

In my practice, a very substantial percentage of my patients have previously undergone spinal fusion (surgical placement of various types of screws and rods to stop instability of the spine). This circumstance doesn't mean you're doomed to chronic pain; most often, complications from surgery can be effectively treated in the hands of a competent interventional orthopedic physician.

When a patient who's had a lumbar surgery comes to our clinic, we look for very specific things related to the surgery. In patients who've had a laminectomy (simple decompression with removal of a small portion of the bone to access the epidural space) and diskectomy (removal of the herniated portion of the disc), we're looking for a recurrence of the herniation, and possibly for scar tissue that's formed around the nerve root.

A recurrent herniation without significant scar tissue is treated as though it occurred without any previous surgery. Scar tissue can often be treated through a combination of injection techniques and neural stretching techniques, as would be demonstrated to you by a skilled physical therapist.

After lumbar fusion surgery, the key is to determine whether the fusion was successful. Most often, it was — and then we're looking for pain at the adjacent segments. For fusions that extend from any segment of the lumbar spine continuously through to the sacrum, the pain will usually be in the sacroiliac joints below the fusion and/or in the segment above the fusion.

For fusions performed in isolated segments or only from L4-L5, the most common level of pain will be below the fusion at the level of L5-S1 and possibly in the sacroiliac joints. As with all non-postsurgical lower back pain, we start with physical therapy to focus on voluntary active neutral alignment of the lumbar spine, as well as posture, behavior, strength, flexibility, and overall conditioning.

More often than not, though, these postsurgical patients will have significant secondary problems such as facet joint or sacroiliac joint pain that can be treated effectively with radiofrequency ablation. We've found that most of these patients will have a successful outcome when the basic tenets of our treatment protocol are adhered to. To review, these tenets are as follows:

1. Achieve a specific diagnosis through advanced imaging, physical exam, and/or diagnostic injection techniques.

2. Focus treatment on appropriate modification of posture and behavior, with retraining to help the patient actively and consciously achieve a neutral spinal alignment.

3. Use injection techniques (up to and including ablation techniques and regenerative interventions) as a tool to facilitate rehabilitation.

So if you've had surgery that never relieved your pain or surgery that helped at first but led to recurrent or new pain, don't despair. Help is available!

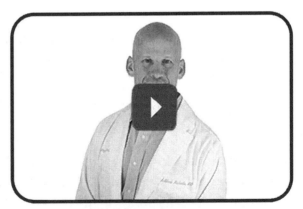

For **Free Video Information**
On This Subject Go To
*whydoihavebackpain.com*

# CHAPTER 10

# Learn the emerging role of regenerative interventions (a potential game-changer)

Over the last several years, we've seen the emergence of biological regenerative treatments such as platelet-rich plasma injections, autologous stem cell injections, and products like Amniofix.

The literature in this field is growing rapidly, and we've seen significant benefit for spinal regenerative therapies. These therapies are very important and will likely become more so as the years go by. There are many people with fragile discs, either through genetics or prior injury, who need to do something to "turn back the clock."

These regenerative procedures are for people who've had disc problems that don't respond adequately to the advice given here. For those individuals, regenerative interventions can be helpful in strengthening the disc and other structures.

Modern regenerative techniques are often criticized for the lack of evidence that they are effective — but it's important to recognize that the evidence of the short- and long-term effectiveness of the most common procedures performed today (including lumbar decompression and lumbar fusion) is equivocal at best. In other words, it's not as though we use regenerative techniques even though there is clear evidence that conventional techniques are more effective.

An additional concern for most people, when it comes to regenerative techniques is that insurance does not pay for them and, therefore, they are an out-of-pocket expense for the patient. In our clinic, as in any other, this is a significant factor. For this reason, we make every effort to start with conventional interventions that insurance will customarily pay for. Most of our patients will get better this way without any non-covered procedures. A conversation about regenerative techniques will occur when the patient asks — or when all conventional options have been exhausted and the patient is still having significant loss of function related to pain. The details of these regenerative techniques will be discussed in a forthcoming book.

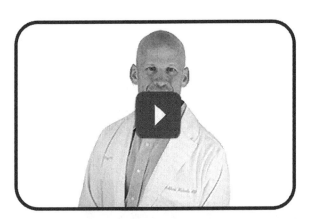

For **Free Video Information**
On This Subject Go To
***whydoihavebackpain.com***

Made in the USA
Lexington, KY
25 November 2017